The 5 Biological Laws

Anxiety and Panic Attacks

Dr. Hamer's New Medicine

The 5 Biological Laws Anxiety and Panic Attacks

Dr. Hamer's New Medicine

ISBN-13: 978-1530113316

ISBN-10: 1530113318

Publisher: Createspace

For information and orders of the following book, you can contact the Author by following addresses:

www.5biologicallaws.com

The relative medical discoveries to the Germanic New Medicine® are protected by copyright inside the books published by Amici di Dirk®, and they belong to the same Dr. Mag. Theol. Ryke Geerd Hamer.

to Matilde

Warnings

The author declines any responsibility for the information and use of the matters treated in this text. Nothing here stated wants to replace the academic and official medicine.

Nowadays, the discoveries of Dr. Hamer are not verified and recognized by the Official Medicine yet.

I remember to the reader that this text doesn't want to replace some diagnosis and medical therapy, but the same is addressed to competent therapists to compare the benefits, and the risks of the therapies offered for the time being.

Andrea Taddei

The 5 Biological Laws

Anxiety and Panic Attacks

Dr. Hamer's New Medicine

Index

PRESENTATION   13

1. DR. HAMER'S NEW MEDICINE   15

2. THE 5 BIOLOGICAL LAWS   17
    1st Biological Law of Nature   17
    2rd Biological Law of Nature   21
    3rd Biological Law of Nature   27
    4th Biological Law of Nature   29
    5th Biological Law of Nature   33

2. BIOLOGICAL CONFLICTS   35
    "Morsel" conflicts   37
    "Attack" conflicts *(or fear of being attacked)* 39
    "self-devaluation" Conflicts   40
    "Territory and separation" conflicts   41

3. THE "CONFLICT ACTIVE" PHASE   43

4. CONFLICTOLYSIS   47

5. POST-CONFLICTOLYSIS PHASE   49

6. A CHANGE OF PERSPECTIVE   57

7. LATERALITY   61

8. HANGING HEALINGS   63

9. CONFLICT RELAPSES OR "TRACKS"   65

10. REFUGEE CONFLICT   67

11. THE CEREBRAL CONSTELLATIONS   71

12. ANXIETY AND PANIC ATTACKS   75

APPENDIX   91
    The Nervous System   91

CHARTS   97

ABOUT THE AUTHOR   105

BIBLIOGRAPHY   107

Presentation

The New Germanic Medicine® discovered by the Dr. Ryke Geerd Hamer and systematized in the five Biological Laws, it represents a change in the understanding of what is commonly called "Illness".

Through his studies, Dr. R. G. Hamer, has reached the ascertainment that the pathological courses are not "errors of the nature" but, on the contrary, Sensible Biological Programs of the Nature consequent on sudden and dramatic events.

This book, in the context of the five Biological Laws, has been written with the intent to carry out a greater understanding on the origin and the meaning, from the biologic point of view, of the anxiety and the panic attack.

1. Dr. Hamer's New Medicine

According to the German Doctor Ryke Geerd Hamer, the cause of the illnesses must be found in "particular events" that the individual lives during his existence. By his studies, started following the loss of his child Dirk and lasted several years, he reached the conclusion the beginning of what we commonly call "illness" is represented by a dramatic and unexpected event the individual suffers, and that he has called "Syndrome of Dirk Hamer" (DHS).

Thanks to his research, he has allowed to redefine radically the concept of illness, not just only as a "mistake of the nature" but on the contrary, as part of a biological programme that has origins in reply to a particular biological-conflictual event; he has discovered and verified that there is a relationship between what a person lives and what has always been defined and considered as "illness". Initially, the Dr. Hamer thought about having found the cause of the cancer, but soon he ascertained that his conclusions could be applied to all the courses that always have been defined for a long time as "pathological". When a person lives an unexpected biological shock, an activation of a precise cerebral area occurs, and this is in univocal relationship to a specific peripheral tissue, organ or bowel, that will give a symptomatic demonstration in a certain moment (symptom) and the so-called "illness".

Thanks to the five Biological Laws it is possible to explain the logic by which the nature of the organism responds to particular events, and consequently, these biological laws bring us to understand the genesis of the illnesses.

Besides this, according to this vision, we can both know the reason why it originates one "illness", and it is also possible to understand its course in the time and in a determined individual in comparison to another. The grandeur of this discovery is that every single law is verifiable by whoever and for any symptom in the totality of the cases.

2. The 5 Biological Laws

1st Biological Law of Nature

1st Criterion: every Significant Biological Special Programs of Nature (SBS) originates from DHS (Dirk Hamer Syndrome), with an unexpected conflict shock, acute and dramatic, lived intensely and with a feeling of isolation. Starting from DHS, every SBS manifests itself simultaneously on three levels: psyche, brain, organ.

2nd Criterion: DHS determines the location of the SBS both at brain level, the so-called Hamer Focus, and at organ level where it causes an organic alteration.

3rd Criterion: the course of the SBS runs synchronously on all three levels (psyche, brain and organ), from DHS to the resolution of the conflict (CL), including epi-crisis (CE) at the top of the Post-Conflict phase (PCL) until normal level is restored (normotonia).

As shown in the picture, we have a line that represents time passing by: it can be shown in seconds, minutes, hours, days, months or years, according to the shock occurred.

time →

Above this line the sympathetic nervous system - also called orthosympathetic - is shown. (see Appendix)

Sympathicotonia

t →

Under the timeline the parasympathetic nervous system is shown.

t →

Vagotonia

Usually we are in a status of normotonia.

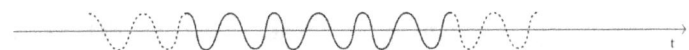

That is to say we physiologically fluctuate from a sympathetic nervous system activation to the parasympathetic nervous system activation: it is the day-night rhythm and the rest-activity rhythm.

During this normotonia - this is quite normal- an acute, unexpected, sudden, dramatic event may occur, which catches me off-guard and I live it as a state of isolation.

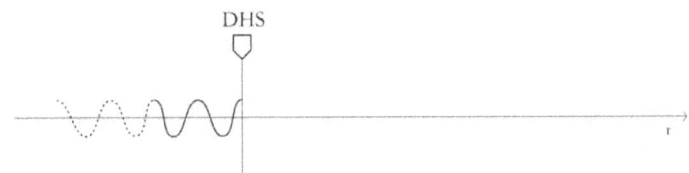

This event (DHS) represents the beginning of a cascade of immediate modifications that will occur simultaneously and instantly at three levels: at a psychic level I will have the memory of the biological conflict (DHS), at brain level, there will be an activation of the cerebral areas (HH-Hamer Focus) that are connected to the event experienced, while at an organ or bowel level, there will be some functional and structural modifications still connected to the event.

The DHS is a biological and not a psychological event.

The living organism should react in an optimal way and straight away to this event, as there is a risk for its safety, its own existence or the existence of the group to which it belongs.

2rd Biological Law of Nature

All Special Programs with the Biological Sense(SBS) consist of two phases, provided that you get to the solution of the conflict.

The 2nd Biological Law describes the Significant Biological Special Programs of Nature (SBS) : the bi-phasic state of the sympaticotonia/parasympaticotonia following the biological conflict (DHS) experienced by the individual at a given moment and it is marked by a series of specific events:

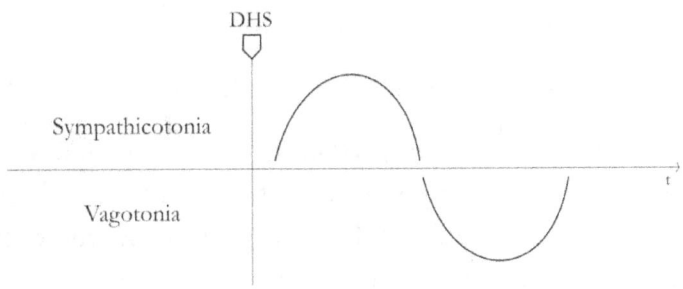

Since DHS has occurred, following a fully meaningful logic from a biological point of view, one can see an activation of the orthosympathetic nervous system: this activation is absolutely optimal to allow the individual to react to that sudden, unexpected event that has caught him off-guard.

The activation of the ortosympathetic system will last until the initial conflict is resolved (DHS). This status of sympathicotonia can be more or less intense (shock mass) depending on the type of conflict experienced. Throughout the sympaticotonia status there will be physic and psychic signs that will show one is in a Conflict-Active phase (CA):

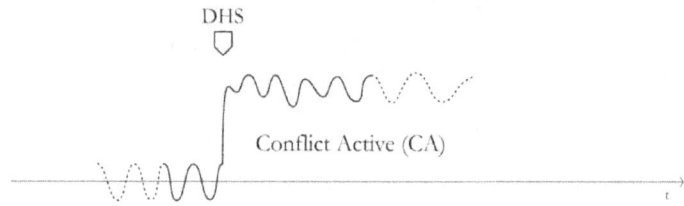

On a psyche level, the person will continue to think about what has happened (obsessive thought), day and night (if it has been particularly intense): this is due to the activation of the sympathethic nervous system.

On a vegetative level, the person will have cold hands and feet, cold skin, lack of appetite, weight loss, insomnia with awakenings between 1 and 3 am and hyperactivity; all this is due to the constant stimulation of the sympathethic nervous system.

On a cerebral level, there will be the formation of the so called Hamer Foci (HH) in specific areas related to the experienced conflict and the corresponding organ. These can be seen during a CAT/CT scan (computerized axial tomography) without contrast.

On an organic level, there will be a structural and functional modification, depending on the embryological origin of the tissue being stimulated by the sympathetic system (3rd Biological Law). During the Active Conflict phase, there are no symptoms (with notably rare exceptions).

This sympathicotonia status following the DHS allows the individual to be able to resolve the conflict in good time (days, weeks or months) and if it happens, this is called Conflictolysis (CL):

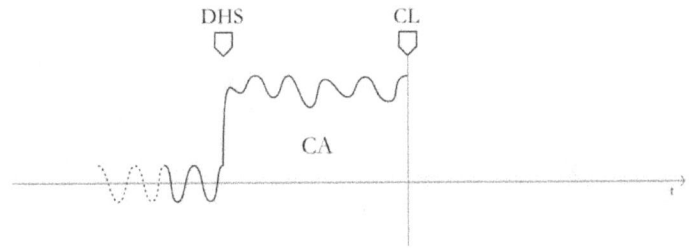

Conflictolysis marks the transition to a second phase, opposite to the first, where there is an activation of the parasympathethic nervous system or vagotonia.

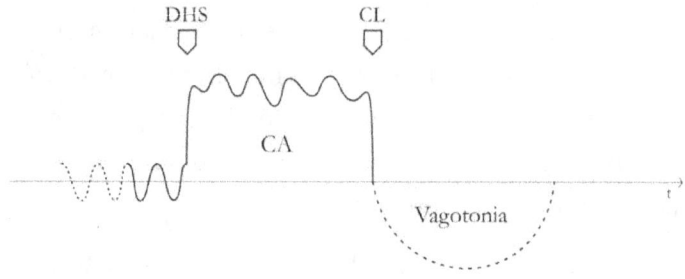

This second vagotonic phase is composed of a phase called A (PCL-A Post-Conflictolysis A), a sympathicotonic phase or peak (Epileptoid Crisis, CE) and a phase B (PCL-B or Post-Conflictolysis B). The duration of this phase is related to the duration of the Conflict-Active phase:

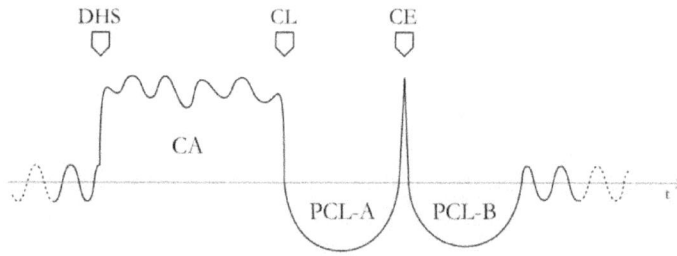

"Just to allow the reader to understand the performance of the 2nd Biological Law discovered by Dr.Hamer, I have reproduced here the biphasic curve chart which partly calls to mind the original by Dr.Hamer as reported in Bibliography."

Throughout the vagotonic status, I will have physic and psychic symptoms that will indicate that I am in a PCL (Post-Conflictolysis) status, also called Healing Phase.

On a psyche level, one will no longer think of the event occurred, as this is now settled and remote, and one will be very calm.

On a vegetative level, one will have: warm hands and feet, fatigue.

On a cerebral level, the so-called Hamer-Focus (HF) will show a different conformation of the specific areas related to the experienced conflict and the corresponding organ. These can be seen during a CAT scan (computerized axial tomography) without contrast.

On an organic level, there will be a structural and functional modification,it being the opposite of the sympathicotonic phase one (3rd Biological Law). At this stage, signs and physical symptoms appear, which are precisely related to the DHS suffered previously.

3rd Biological Law of Nature

The ontogenetically conditioned system of the Significant Biological Special Programs of Nature (SBS)

Each tissue originally stems from one of the three embryonic germ layers called: Endoderm, Mesoderm (old and new), Ectoderm (see Appendix); every single tissue derived from a specific embryonic germ layer is subject to a stimulation of the autonomic nervous system (sympathicotonia-parasympathicotonia) and can be subject to one of the four different structural and functional alterations:

- tissue increase (proliferation)

- tissue reduction (necrosis, ulceration)

- increased tissue function (hyperfunction)

- reduced tissue function (hypofunction)

All the tissues that are derived from Endoderm, in the sympathicotonic phase (CA) will have a tissue and function increase, while in the parasympaticotonic phase (PCL) they will have a loss of function and tissue:

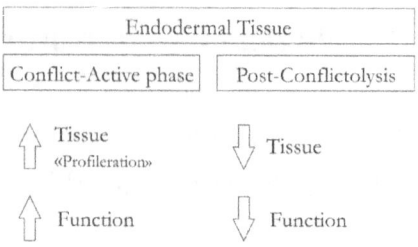

All the tissues that derive from Old Mesoderm, in the sympathicotonic phase (CA) will show a loss of tissue and function, while in the parasympathicotonic phase (PCL)they will show an increase of function and tissue:

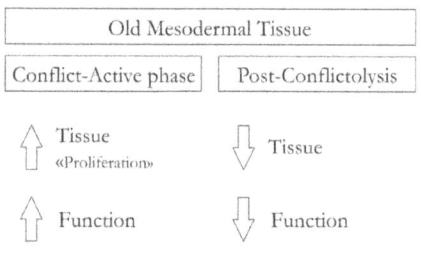

All the tissues deriving from New Mesoderm, in the sympathicotonic phase (CA) will have a loss of tissue and function, while in the parasympathicotonic phase (PCL) they will have an increase of function and tissue:

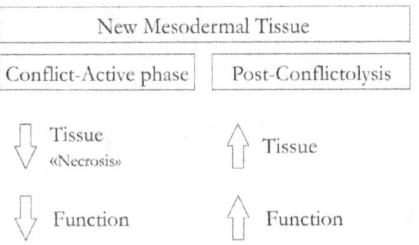

All the tissues that come from Ectoderm, in the sympathicotonic phase (CA) face a loss of tissue and function, while in the parasympathicotonic phase (PCL) they face an increase of function and tissue:

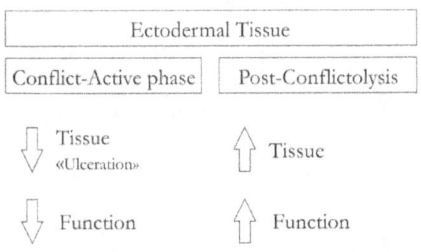

4th Biological Law of Nature

The genetically determined microbial system in the History of Evolution.

Fungi, bacteria and viruses are actively involved in the 2nd phase of the bi-phasic curve (PCL), optimizing the resolution phase.

Endodermal Tissue	Mesodermal Tissue	Ectodermal Tissue

Fungi, Mycobacteria

Bacteria

Virus

The **Fungi and Mycobacteria** (TBC) participate in the reduction of the tissue deriving from Endoderm that in the active phase (CA) was increased or they do a caseification only during the post-conflict phase. The mycobacteria can also be found in some tissues derived from Old Mesoderm.

The **Bacteria** that derive from Mesoderm proliferate in the active phase (CA) and optimize the tissue healing phase (PCL)

The **Viruses** are in the tissues that derive from Ectoderm in PCL phase and optimize the reconstruction process, restoring the structure.

5th Biological Law of Nature

The quintessence

The 5th biological law reminds us that the Significant Biological Special Programs of Nature (SBS) activated with a DHS have a specific biological sense to ensure the survival of the individual or of the group.

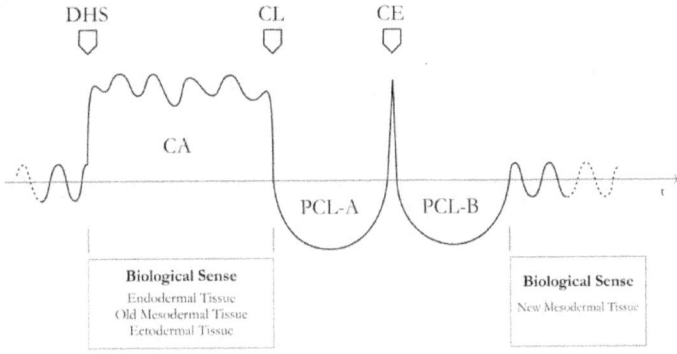

The biological sense is for all tissues in the Active Conflict phase, except for tissues that derive from the New Mesoderm, directed by the White Matter, in which it occurs at the end of the healing phase (normotonia).

2. Biological conflicts

Among all the events that a person experiences, only some will represent a DHS. These are all those conflicts in which the following conditions occur:

- unexpected

- sudden

- acute

- dramatic

- experienced in isolation

They are called Biological Conflicts as the occurring event represents a "biological difficulty" which the individual has to overcome and respond to, in order to ensure its biological integrity, survival or integrity of the group to which it belongs.

The reaction is automatic, immediate, instinctive and not mediated by ego; only these conflicts can be called biological and are the only ones that will allow to start the Significant Special Biological Program (SBS); completely different from those conflicts, in Psychology, in which conflict is a clash between what a person desires and his/her inner/interpersonal needs and this clash doesn't allow the satisfaction of this desire, of the need itself or of the objective related to that desire: these are certainly inconveniences for the individual, but will not be capable of causing the activation of a Significant Biological Special Program.

The biological conflicts that can issue a DHS, are the following:

- "Morsel" conflicts
- "Attack" conflicts *(or fear of being attacked)*
- "Self-devaluation" conflicts
- "Territory and separation" conflicts

Only these conflicts and only if experienced as DHS by the individual (unexpected, sudden, dramatic and lived in isolation) will cause functional and tissue alterations as a significant answer, following the trend of the biphasic curve and the 3rd Biological Law.

Conflicts and the Significant Biological Special Program (SBS) that are produced, allow us both as individuals and as a species to survive in worst-case scenarios and in less dramatic cases to react to the unexpected occurred event.

"Morsel" conflicts

These conflicts are related to the survival of the individual, of his species and the maintenance of vital functions: eating, digesting, assimilating, eliminating, evacuating, breathing, hearing and reproduction.

The morsel conflict, with all its variants, involves all the tissues that derive from Endoderm, that is to say from that embryonic germ layer directly involved in preserving the body's vital functions; these are the tissues:

- Oral Submucosa
- Palate
- Parotid Glands
- Sublingual Salivary Glands
- Tonsils
- Naso-Pharynx
- Lacrimal glands
- Iris
- Thyroid Gland
- Neurohypophysis
- Middle ear
- Eustachian tube
- Esophagus *(lower third only)*
- Lung alveoli
- Stomach *(greater curvature only)*
- Duodenum *(except for duodenal bulb)*
- Liver parenchyma *(no bile ducts nor cholecyst)*

- Pancreas parenchyma *(except for pancreatic ducts and Langerhans islets)*
- Small and Large Intestine *(Colon)*
- Tongue
- Sigmoid and Rectum *(upper third)*
- Bladder
- Kidney Collecting Tubules
- Prostate
- Uterus and Fallopian Tubes
- Bartholin's glands
- Smegma glands
- Inner navel
- Nuclei of the Acoustic Nerves

The morsel, which is essential for the survival of the individual, is associated to food as well as air morsel (lung alveoli), light morsel (eye, enteroidea), sound morsel (middle ear), water morsel (kidney collecting tubules).

The emotional contents of the morsel conflicts related to man are, to name just a few:

- conflict of "not being able to digest a morsel"
- conflict of "not being able to swallow a morsel"
- death-fright conflict
- conflict of "inability to catch a morsel"
- ...

"Attack" conflicts *(or fear of being attacked)*

These conflicts are related to feeling attacked by everything surrounding the individual, feeling one's own integrity attacked.

The conflict of feeling attacked, with all its variants, involves all tissues that derive from Old Mesoderm, the embryonic germ layer directly concerned with the protection of the individual; these are the tissues:

- Corium Skin *(dermis)*
- Breast Glands (milk producing glands) *(except for ducts)*
- Pericardium *(sac containing the heart)*
- Pleura *(lining of the lungs)*
- Peritoneum *(membrane lining of the abdominal cavity and abdominal organs)*
- Greater Omentum

The emotional contents of Attack conflicts (or fear of being attacked) related to man are, to name just a few:

- Conflict of rejecting contact
- Conflict of attack to one's integrity
- Conflict of personal disfigurement
- Conflict of attack against one's heart
- …

"Self-devaluation" conflicts

These conflicts are related to feeling devaluated, fear of failing, not feeling adequate, not being good at doing something, not being up to scratch.

The self-devaluation conflict, with all its variables, involves all the tissues that derive from New Mesoderm, that is to say that embryonic germ layer involved in the individual's growth and strengthening of the group; these are the derived tissues:

- Bones (including tooth dentin)
- Cartilage
- Tendons and Ligaments
- Connective tissue
- Fat tissue
- Lymphatic system (Lymph vessels & Lymphnodes)
- Blood vessels (except coronary vessels)
- Muscles (striated musculature)
- Myocardium (80% striated heartmuscle)
- Kidney Parenchyma
- Adrenal cortex
- Spleen
- Ovaries
- Testicles

The emotional contents of the devaluation conflicts related to the individual are, to name just a few:

- Conflict of intellectual devaluation
- Conflict of not being adequate
- Conflict of incapability to escape a situation
- Conflict of feeling left outside a situation
- Conflict of having lost someone
- Conflict of being tied to a ball and chain
- …

"Territory and separation" conflicts

These conflicts are related to the group to which one belongs, to the territory and separation. The territorial conflict (fight and separation), with all its variants, involves all tissues that stem from Ectoderm, that is to say that embryonic germ layer directly connected to territorial fight and separation. These are the tissues stemming from the ectoderm:

- Epidermis *(skin)*
- Periosteum *(skin that covers the bones)*
- Mouth *(upper mucosa)*, incl. palate, gums, tongue, lining of salivary gland ducts
- Nasal and sinuses membrane
- Inner ear
- Lens, cornea, conjunctiva, retina, and vitreous body of the eyes
- Teeth enamel
- Lining of the milk ducts

- Lining of the thyroid gland ducts and of pharyngeal ducts
- Lining of the heart vessels *(coronary arteries and coronary veins)*
- Esophagus *(upper 2/3)*
- Laryngeal mucosa and Bronchial mucosa
- Stomach lining *(small curvature)*
- Lining of the bile ducts and gall bladder, and of pancreatic ducts
- Cervix and vagina
- Lining of renal pelvis, bladder, ureter, and urethra
- Lining of the rectum *(lower part)*
- Nerve cells of the Central Nervous System

The emotional contents of territorial conflicts related to man are, to name just a few :

- Territorial conflict
- Territorial threatening conflict
- Territorial anger conflict
- Conflict of inability of marking the territory
- Separation conflict
- Conflict of having no right to bite

For a detailed study of conflicts relating to DHS may the reader refer to the Scientific Table of Germanic New Medicine® (Ed. Amici di Dirk).

3. The "Conflict Active" phase

The DHS that occurred marks the beginning of the Significant Biologic Special program of Nature. The sympathethic nervous system will be activated to bring a response to the event, which occurred so suddenly and unexpectedly, in order to solve it as soon as possible: this phase is called Conflict-Active (CA).

The individual in a Conflict-Active phase will continue to mull all day long over that event that occurred so unexpectedly and, if this event has been very intense, the person will think about it also during the night and wake up between 1 and 3 am. On a somatic level,the individual will have very cold hands and feet, lack of appetite, hyperactivity, mild fatigue.

During the Conflict-Active phase, the individual is fine and has no symptoms that can worry him, all his physical and mental energies are directed to solve his problem (DHS). Other smaller problems are momentarily put aside and, in any case, they are not a priority at this time.

In this phase, depending on the type of conflict (DHS) experienced by the individual, the tissues begin to "respond" to the sympathicotonia status but there are no symptoms:

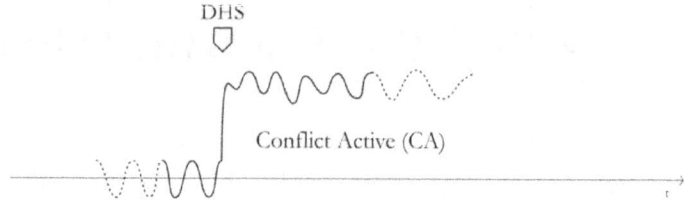

DHS

Conflict Active (CA)

If DHS is related to a morsel conflict corresponding to a tissue that derives from Endoderm, in the Conflict-Active phase, the tissue will increase (proliferation) and its related function will increase as well:

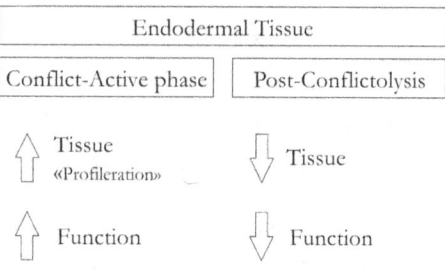

If DHS is related to an attack conflict corresponding to a tissue that derives from Old Mesoderm, in the Conflict-Active phase, the tissue will increase and its related function will increase as well:

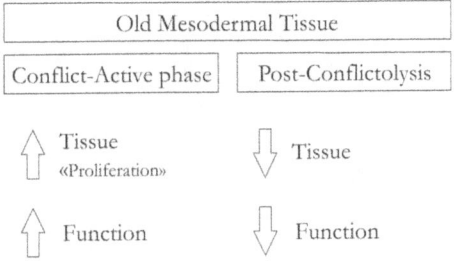

If DHS is related to a self-devaluation conflict corresponding to a tissue that derives from New Mesoderm, in the Conflict-Active phase, the tissue will be reduced and so will its related function:

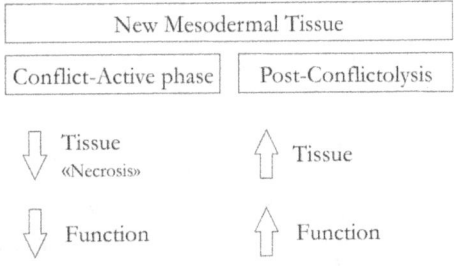

If DHS is related to a territorial conflict corresponding to a tissue that comes from Endoderm, in the Conflict Active phase, the tissue will be reduced (ulceration) and so will its function:

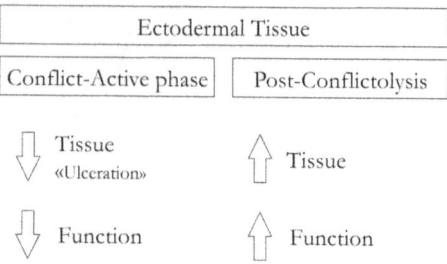

The biological sense (5th Biological Law) for all conflicts that derive from Endoderm, from Old Mesoderm and Ectoderm is in the Conflict-Active phase:

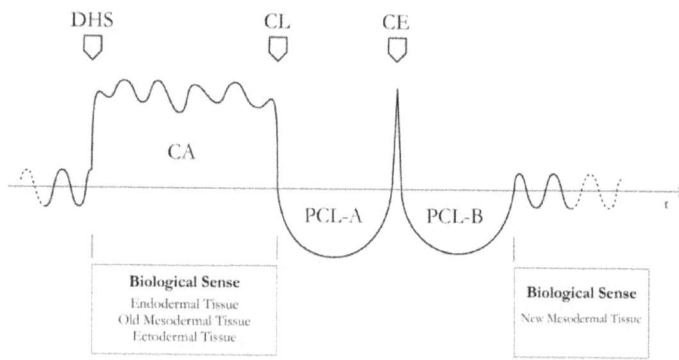

4. Conflictolysis

Conflictolysis occurs when, thanks to the state of sympathicotonia, I have been in, I am able to resolve the conflict (DHS). The resolution of the conflict can happen in different ways, more or less depending on the individual; one can manage to finally get away from what has happened, one can deal with the situation or, it may occur, circumstances spontaneously evolve in a better direction even without one's direct intervention:

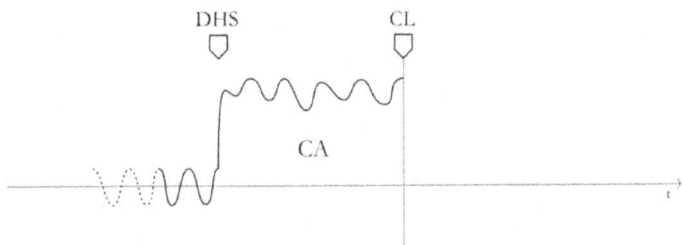

Conflictolysis is an event that allows the resolution of a biological conflict, has a positive connotation, it represents a relief, a solution.

After Conflictolysis, a phase change occurs; from a status of ortosympathicotonia, a parasympathicotonia or vagotonic phase will appear and this is called Post-Conflictolysis phase of resolution.

48

5. Post-Conflictolysis Phase

The Healing phase - Post Conflictolysis (PCL) represents the second phase of the biphasic curve; the autonomic nervous system switches from activation of the sympathetic to an activation of the parasympathetic:

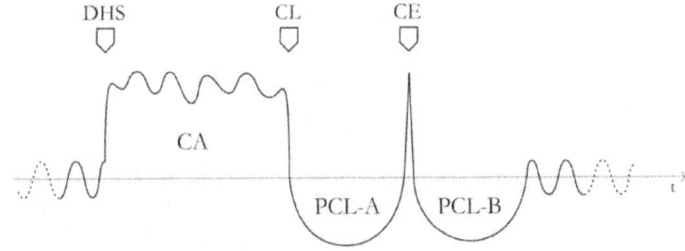

In this vagotonic phase, the individual will be tired and will sleep longer than usual if possible, he will no longer think of his problem because it is finally solved and at a somatic level he will have warm hands, feet and skin and he will see signs and symptoms that will prompt him to a medical consultation to give a name to his "disease".

The symptoms that occur in this phase are related to the type of DHS occurred earlier and which started the Significant Biological Special program: a cold, bronchitis, vitiligo, dermatitis, gastritis, hepatitis, cystitis, psoriasis, pleurisy, conjunctivitis, myopia, low back pain, rhinitis, headache, arthritis… and all the so-called "diseases" that have a precise and unique correspondence with a biological conflict (DHS)

In this second phase called vagotonic, the tissues begin to respond to the parasympathicotonic phase (3rd Biological Law):

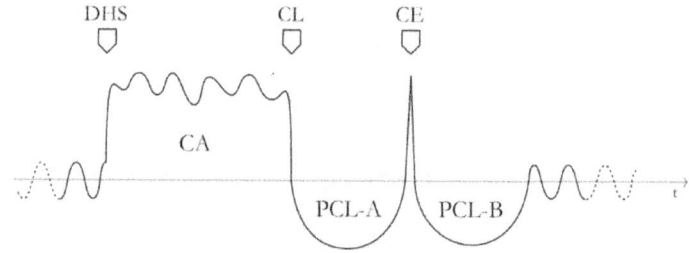

If DHS is related to a morsel conflict, that corresponds to any tissue that derives from Endoderm in resolution, the tissue and its function will be reduced:

Endodermal Tissue	
Conflict-Active phase	Post-Conflictolysis
⇧ Tissue «Profileration»	⇩ Tissue
⇧ Function	⇩ Function

If DHS is related to a attack conflict, that corresponds to any tissue that derives from Old Mesoderm in resolution, the tissue and its function will be reduced:

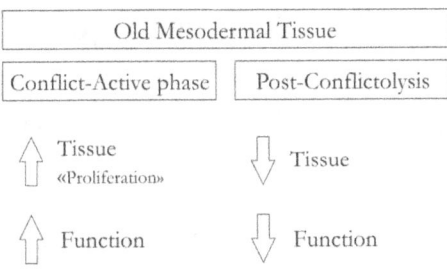

If DHS is related to a devaluation conflict, corresponding to any tissue deriving from the New Mesoderm in resolution, the tissue and its function will end this phase with a surplus of tissue:

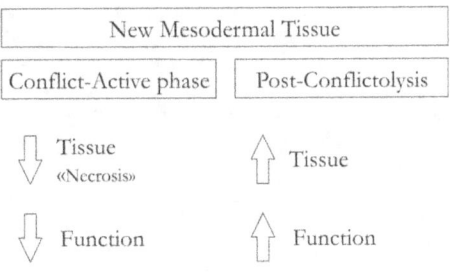

If DHS is related to a territorial conflict, that corresponds to any tissue that derives from Ectoderm in resolution, the tissue and its function will be replenished:

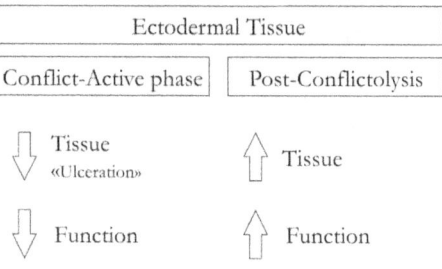

As you can see in this picture, the vagotonic resolution phase is composed by three curves:

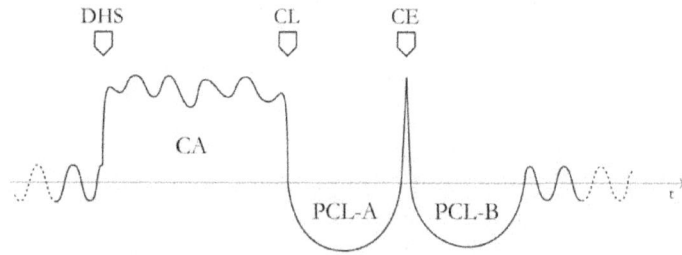

The PCL A (Post-Conflictolysis phase A) is the first parasympathicotonic in which one or more symptoms appear. Analysing a single biphasic curve and without conflict relapses, the temporal duration of this phase is exactly half the duration of the Conflict-Active phase but with a maximum duration of 3 weeks (e.g.):

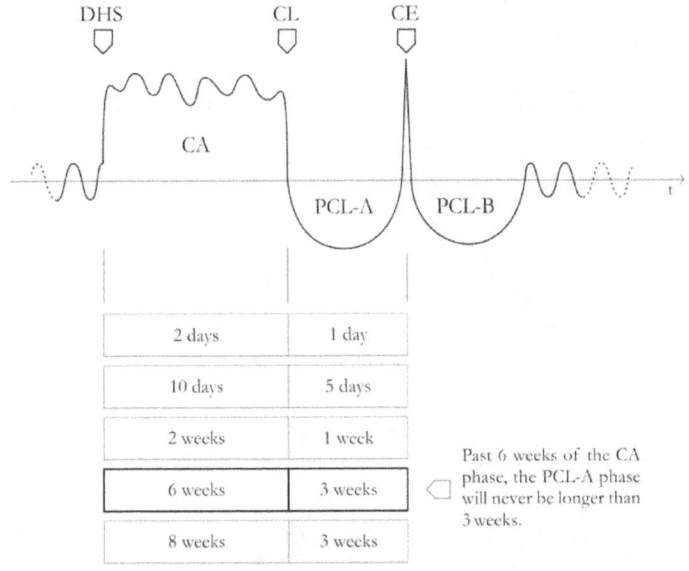

2 days	1 day
10 days	5 days
2 weeks	1 week
6 weeks	3 weeks
8 weeks	3 weeks

Past 6 weeks of the CA phase, the PCL-A phase will never be longer than 3 weeks.

If the CA phase lasted two weeks, the PCL A phase has a duration of one week. Past 6 weeks of the CA phase, the PCL A phase will never be longer than 3 weeks).

After the PCL A phase, a sympathicotonic peak is shown, which is called EPILEPTOID CRISIS (EPI-CRISIS) (CE) (If DHS is motorial, it will be called Epileptic crisis). This sympathicotonic peak occurs in the middle of the healing phase and its function is to reduce the brain edema at the HH level : it will be associated to very intense and acute symptoms called renal colic, biliary colic, intestinal colic, panic attack (and more) but it will always be in relation to the emotional content of the initial DHS.

Biologically, the epi-crysis has a duration that can range from 10 -20 seconds to 4 hours:

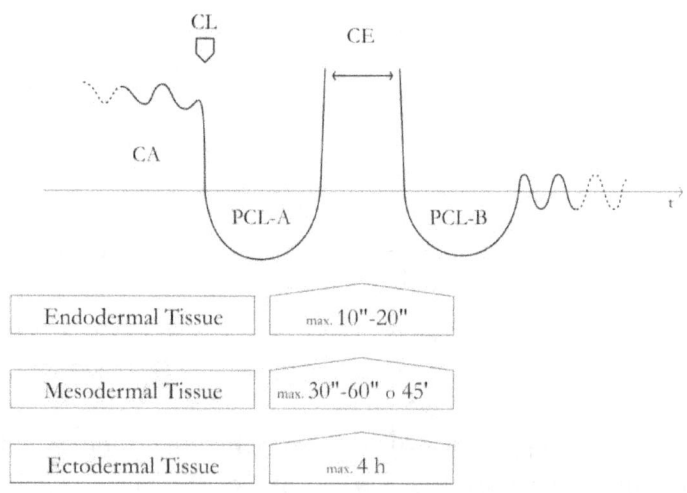

Endodermal Tissue	max. 10"-20"
Mesodermal Tissue	max. 30"-60" o 45'
Ectodermal Tissue	max. 4 h

The duration of the Epi-crysis, it often happens, can exceed maximum if it enters a "hanging" phase.

At the end of the Epileptoid crisis a vagotonic phase will recur, called PCL B, with less intense symptoms, which will mark the end of the Significant Biological special Program of Nature before getting back to normotonia:

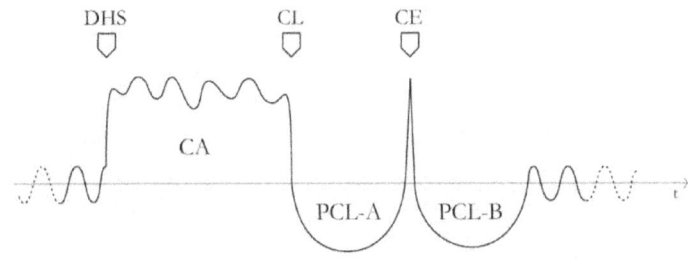

During the Post-Conflictolysis phase, besides having the specific symptoms determined by the DHS and the type of tissue involved, one may also run a temperature of varying degrees, depending on the embryonic derivation of tissue:

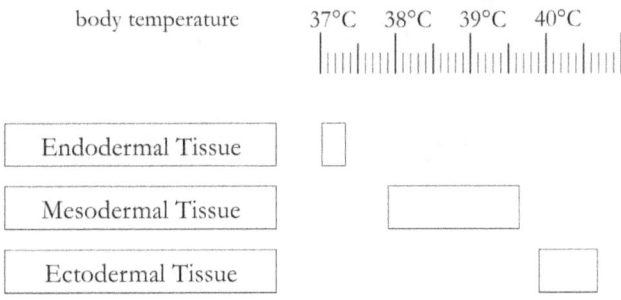

The biological sense (5th Biological Law) for tissues that derive from the new Mesoderm comes at the end of the biphasic curve, when normotonia is restored:

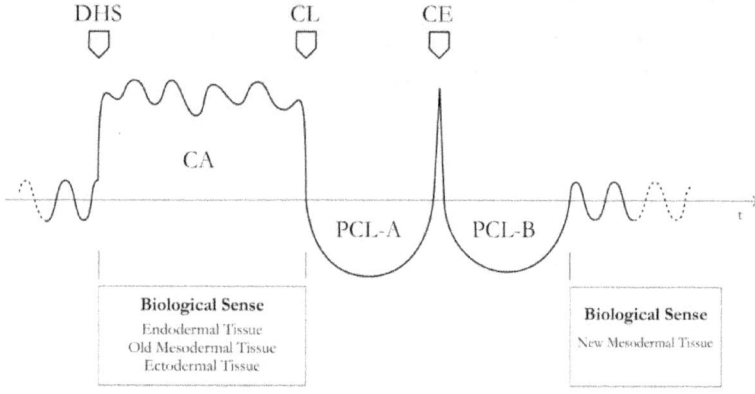

6. A change of perspective

"... at the end I have had to ask myself if our understanding, and our concept of illness had not been totally wrong because of our ignorance of the biological purpose of the illness... "

R.G. Hamer

There is no shade of doubt that the Official Medicine, from the advent of the antibiotic (1930-1941) to our days, has reached incomparable successes, through a scientific approach, in the field of the pharmacological therapy and surgical therapy, in emergency medicine and in the instrumental diagnosis (Radiography, Cat scan, RMN, PET, Endoscopy...).

This type of methodological approach even if correct, it has carried out to study every phenomenon to an extreme level of detail more and more, but it had consequently, caused the loss of a full vision of the individual in his triad: body, mind and spirit.

What it is derived it is an incapability, of the Official Medicine, to discover the cause of the illnesses, to explain the reason why the illness manifests itself in an individual rather than in another, why the proposed therapies, according to the standard protocols, work for some individuals and not in others.

Doctor Ryke Geerd Hamer, owing to arising of one illness of his consequent to a family mourning, started investigating on the patients if there was a correlation among "traumatic events" and the onset of their illnesses; with his great surprise, he ascertained and verified in the years of study that all the so said "Illnesses" from the most banal to the most serious, they were the consequence of certain types of "events" that he called DHS (Syndrome of Dirk Hamer, 1° Biological Law) that the person had lived.

In his studies, he discovered not only the initial event or the cause of the illnesses, but he also discovered the logic of the trend in the time of the so said "pathological courses" (2° Biological Law).

Initially, because of professional bias, he was searching the problem, the mistake causing the beginning of the illness. In time and with his obsessive research, he reached the amazing understanding that the "illnesses" would not be a malignant phenomenon but rather a "sensible biological programme of the nature" with one "function", every time, well precise to guarantee the survival of the individual and the group.

The "illness" itself would be a sensible reaction of the individual in reply to a special case (Biological Conflict). The course is auto-limited in the time, if other factors don't intervene (see: The Relapses) and it would finish bringing the individual back in a state of "physiological normality".

New Germanic Medicine® is not something alternative to the medicine neither a cure nor a therapy, but it can be considered as a new point of view and study of all those courses defined "pathological"; through the five Biological Laws, one can understand and describe in a scientific way, precise and always verifiable, the causes, the symptoms and the evolution of any course considered "pathological".

7. Laterality

It is fundamental to know whether you are right- or left-handed to understand how the individual functions.

Of all the tests that can be done to determine whether you are right-handed or left-handed, Dr. Hamer was able to verify that the only suitable one to establish the exact laterality is the one of applause.

By applauding like in a theater, the hand that beats above gives dominance: the right-handed individual will hit his right hand over the left while the left-handed will hit his left hand over the right one.

In right-handed people, both male and female, the non-dominant side, the left one ,is related to the nest, to their mother and their children or animals.The right side applies to all other figures (father, husband, lover, friend, friends, girl-friends, employer, in-laws ...):

RIGHT HANDED PEOPLE	
Body Left	Body Right
mother their children animals	father husband, lover, friend, friends, girl- friends, employer, in-laws

In left-handed people,both male and female, the non-dominant side, the right one,is in relation to their mother and their children, or animals, while the dominant regards all other persons:

LEFT HANDED PEOPLE	
Body Left	Body Right
father husband, lover, friend, friends, girl-friends, employer, in-laws	mother their children animals

The rule of laterality applies only to tissues that derive from Mesoderm and Ectoderm.

8. Hanging healings

When a DHS occurs, the individual goes from a Conflict-Active phase (CA) to a Conflictolysis and then a vagotonic Post-Conflictolysis phase starts and will return, with its biologic time, to a normotonia.

We call it "hanging healing" when the individual, instead of progressing to the biphasic curve, as described, will keep going from one vagotonic phase (PCL) to a sympathicotonic one (CA), not necessarily returning to normotonia.

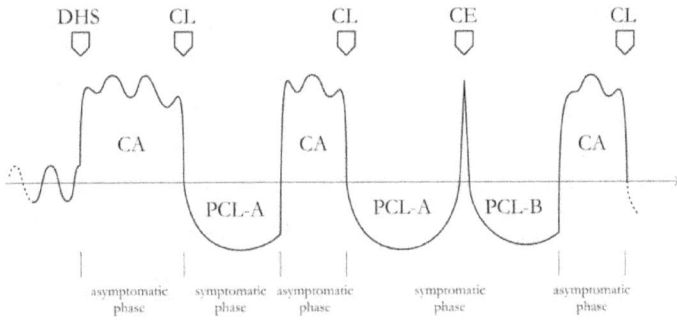

This pattern is due to the fact that, when one is in a vagotonic phase of CA, the event occurs again bringing one back into a conflict-active phase. This trend can last long, even for months.

As to symptoms, they will show in a vagotonic phase (PCL) and then one will experience a fading or disappearance of symptoms in the sympathycotonic phase (CA).

9. Conflict Relapses or "Tracks"

At the exact time DHS occurs, our nervous system records not only the conflict that will trigger the Significant Biologic Special Program but also all those "signals" that accompanied the DHS.

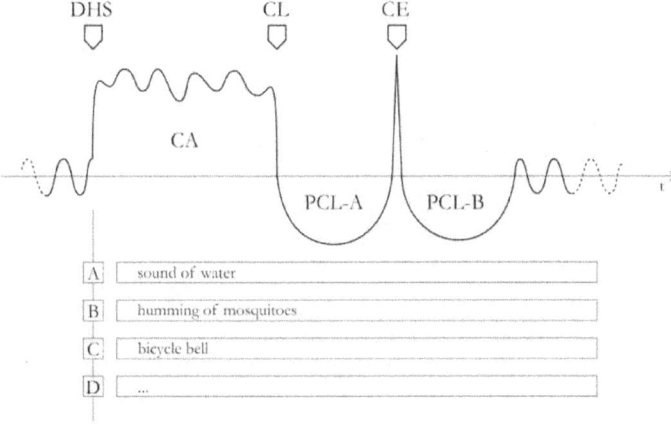

If a DHS of any kind occurs while I am walking on a riverside, in addition to the DHS I will fix a series of "signs", for example, the sound of water, the humming of mosquitoes , the local temperature, the bicycle bell and so on.

These "signals" in future, if reappearing all together or isolated from one another, will reactivate the original biphasic curve related to the event previously experienced years before; if this occurs, as an effect, I will see symptoms showing in relation to the curve.

This mode, from a biological point of view, is optimal because it is a "warning signal" to prevent one from bumping into such a peculiar situation that has already occurred.

10. Refugee Conflict

Whenever one experiences DHS, a new Biological Program(SBS) begins, so if one has different DHS at the same time, one will have different bi-phasic curves, some in an active phase and some in resolution:

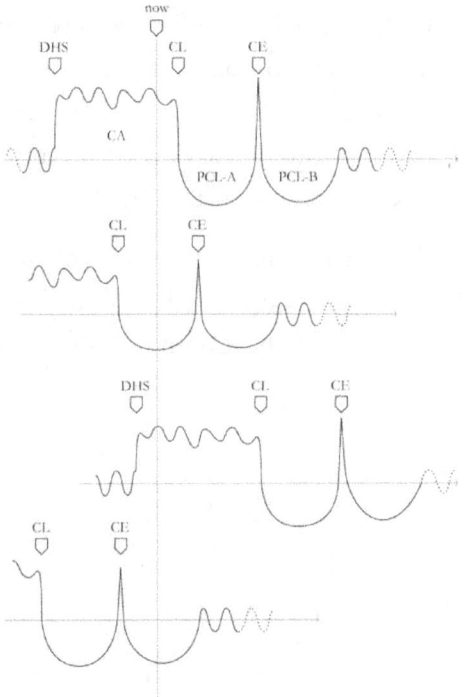

This means that, in a given moment, one will be in CA for one or more DHS, in PCL-A for one or more DHS and in PCL-B for one or more other DHS.

So: for the conflicts I will be having in CA, I will show no symptoms but I will not sleep at night and will feel anxiety.

Instead, I will have a particularly annoying symptom about the conflict in the PCL A phase and a different symptom for the PCL B phase of the DHS that I am living, but at least for this latter conflict in the solution phase I am much calmer and the worst is over.

Among all the biological conflicts we are having, there is a very important and essential one, for its practical implications that can increase, if it is active, the symptomatic manifestation of the parasympatheticotonic curve (PCL-A and B) as well as of any bi-phasic curve related to an active SBS.

This is the refugee conflict, a program of water retention, related to the system of kidney collecting tubules (derivating from Endoderm) that in the Conflict-Active phase, increase their function:

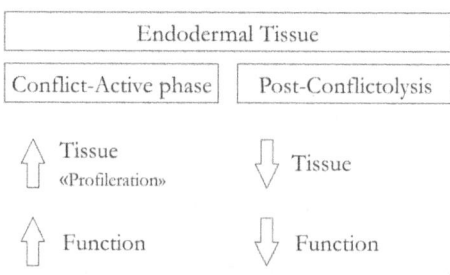

During the sympathicotonic phase of the kidney collecting tubules:

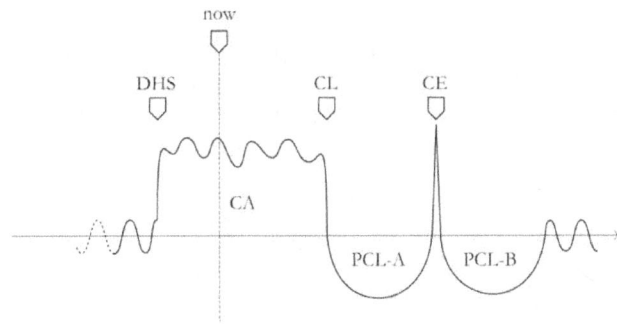

I will experience systemic water retention (the whole body will feel bloated): I will feel bloated, not necessarily with other symptoms, but if in addition to the SBS of collecting tubules(active refugee conflict) I also have another SBS in a solution A phase (PCL-A), the symptoms of this conflict will increase exponentially.

The result will be a local edema of the 2nd curve plus global edema (CA of the kidney collecting tubules) of the 1st curve and this will cause more serious symptoms (local edema + global edema = more pain or symptom):

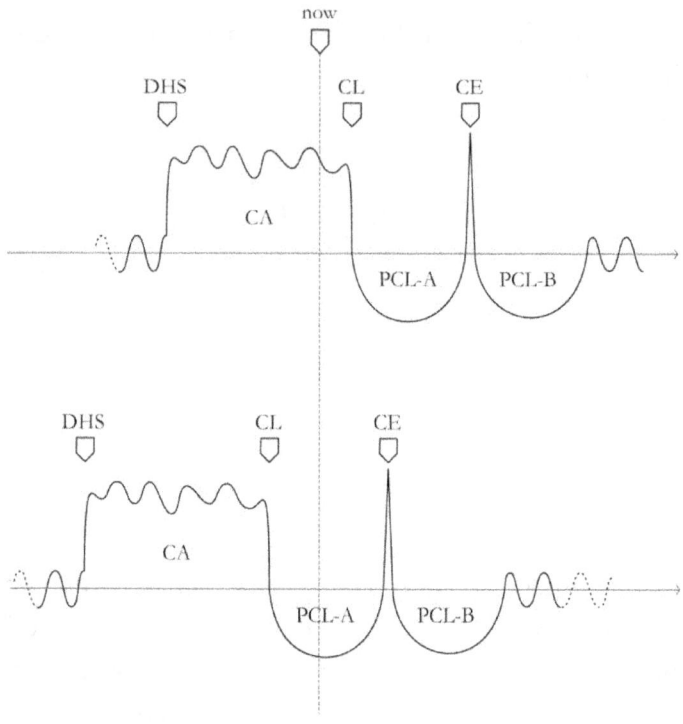

A single healing curve (PCL) gives an ache or a symptom that can reach 2-3 in a range from 1 to 10. Together with an active refugee conflict, the ache goes up to 9-10.

11. The Cerebral Constellations

Dr. Hamer's research has shown how the behavior of the individual develops and follows the same biological laws that explain the physical symptoms, the illnesses; as well as the "mental illnesses" like the depression, the psychoses, the manias, the obsessions, eating disorder like bulimia, anorexia, they have a psychic, cerebral and organic correlation according to the five Biological Laws.

In his research he has been able to understand and verify that when some DHSs occur, corresponding Cerebral Relays are cerebrally activated (1° Biological Law), and if the active relays are cerebrally and contemporarily present both to the right and to the left in the same cerebral area (Trunk, Cerebellum, White substance or Cortex), the individual falls into the so said "Schizophrenic Constellation", or he will show a certain type of "behavior" typical of that activated constellation. The gravity of the "psychic trouble" is always in relation to the intensity and duration of the conflicts that are manifesting (conflictual mass), of other factors (conflict of the tubules' renal collectors).

The constellations manifest when two conflicts are contemporarily in active phase, when one is in active phase (CA) and one in epileptoid crisis (CE) or when both are in epileptoid crisis. There is the exception of the constellations of the cerebral white substance (connected to the devaluation of oneself), where the state of constellation remains also in the parasympathetic post-conflict lytic stage.

Every cerebral area, brain trunk, cerebellum, white substance and cerebral cortex have the relative constellations, let's see some of them:

- **Dismay**: at Cerebral trunk level, center of the relays corresponding to all the tissues deriving from the endoderm, and concerning the conflicts related to the "bit", for example, when a DHS at the stomach level (right portion of the Cerebral Trunk) and a DHS at the bowel level (left portion of the trunk) occur, the resulting constellation will be the "Dismay"; the individual will appear confused, and the ability of reaction and the orientation will be more or less jeopardized.

- **Emotional death**: at the Cerebellum level, where the relative relays and some tissues coming from mesoderm are present (ancient mesoderm) and related to the conflicts of "feeling oneself attacked" the result of a double conflict, cerebrally active both to the right and to le left, will·cause an "emotional death". The individual will feel "emotionally dull", incapable to feel emotions with an asocial behavior.

- **Maniac-depressive constellation**: the cerebral relays of the conflicts that allow "to activate" this constellation; they are found in the insular area, and they are related to the territory and affective-sexual conflicts. According to the "importance" of the conflict, even if other factors can intervene, accentuating the importance more to the right or to the left (cerebrally) the person will show maniacal or depressive manners.

- **Aggressive constellation**: the conflicts of this constellation are related to the conflict of identity (rectal mucous) and to the conflict of grudge of territory (small bending of the stomach, bile, pancreas ducts). If the conflict of identity is more accentuated in comparison to the conflict of grudge of territory, the person can have some explosions of violence toward the others, while contrarily the individual will show hostile manners toward himself (self-injury).

- **Asthmatic constellation**: furthermore, the asthma is part of the cerebral constellations. The involved relays are related to the musculature of the larynx, with the relative conflict of sudden fear and to the bronchial musculature with the relative conflict of the threat of territory. At a practical level, there can be three types of asthma:

- *Bronchial asthma,* the characteristic of this type of asthma is that the person will find hard to expire (prolonged expiration) during the asthmatic attack. This is caused by the fact that the relay related to the bronchial musculature is in Epileptoid Crisis (CE), while the relay related to the pharynx musculature is in Active Conflict (CA).

- *Laryngeal Asthma,* the characteristic of this other type of asthma is that the person will find hard to inhale (prolonged inspiration) during the asthmatic attack. This is caused by the fact that the relay related to the laryngeal musculature is in Epileptoid Crisis (CE), while the relay related to the musculature of the bronchus is in Active Conflict (CA).

- *Asthmatic State,* in this acute state, very serious and requiring for an urgent medical intervention, there is the severe difficulty to breathe both in inspiration and in expiration. Both the relays are contemporarily in Epileptoid Crisis (CE).

Besides these cerebral constellations, shortly exposed, there are other like: Frontal Constellation, Bio-maniacal, Megalomaniac Constellation, Mythomaniac, Occipital, Auditory, Thalamic Bulimic, Anorexic, Obsessive, Motor, Sensory, Post-deadly, Diabetic… if thinking that in the same individual, there could be more constellations activated at the same time, about ten combinations result with different peculiar and behavioral manners.

12. Anxiety and Panic Attacks

The understanding of the five Biological Laws is fundamental to contextualize and organize in the best way, both the anxiety and the panic attacks in relationship to the biphasic curve or to the Biological and Sensible Program of the Nature (2° Biological Law).

The Anxiety

Many people agree that anxiety represents a physiological condition, a fundamental resource, effective in many moments of life to maintain the alert, to help us to find a solution, to protect ourselves from the risks, to improve the answers and the performances in the study, in the job and sport.

Anxiety is a normal phenomenon that involves a state of activation of the neurovegetative system (Autonomous Nervous System) that activates when we live a dangerous situation.

The neurovegetative phenomenons, manifesting during the state of anxiety, are individual and can be various: perspiration, cold and wet hands, tachycardia, dry mouth, nausea, intestinal troubles, burst of heat," lump in the throat", dizziness, muscular tensions, nervousness, incapability to keep still, restlessness, having "the nerves on the edge", irritability, difficulty of concentration, short memory, restless sleep, unsatisfactory or difficulty to fall asleep, obsessive thought.

Such phenomenons are all referable to an activation of the Autonomous Nervous System and more precisely to the activation of the Orthosympathetic System that at a biphasic curve level (SBS) corresponds to the Active Conflict:

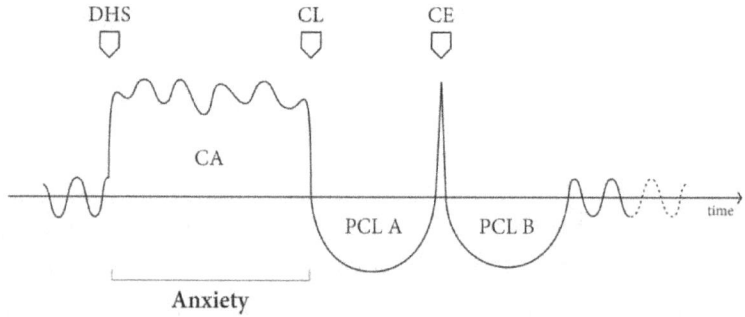

The anxiety, as already said, is a physiological condition that allows the organism to be reactive, to run away, to attack, to react in the most effective way possible, sheltering ourselves and guaranteeing the possibility to survive in a hostile environment.

If the activation is excessive in comparison to the situations we live, one will talk about "trouble of anxiety" and it will become a factor that can complicate the life of a person who is put under the conditions to be incapable to face the most common daily situations, at school, at work, in the relationships.

In this case, according to the five Biological Laws, this type of "excessive reply" is caused by the concomitant activation of the Refugee (see: cap. The Refugee's conflict) that exasperates the intensity of the anxiety.

Anxiety, consequently, manifests itself the most in a precise situation that the individual lives (DHS):

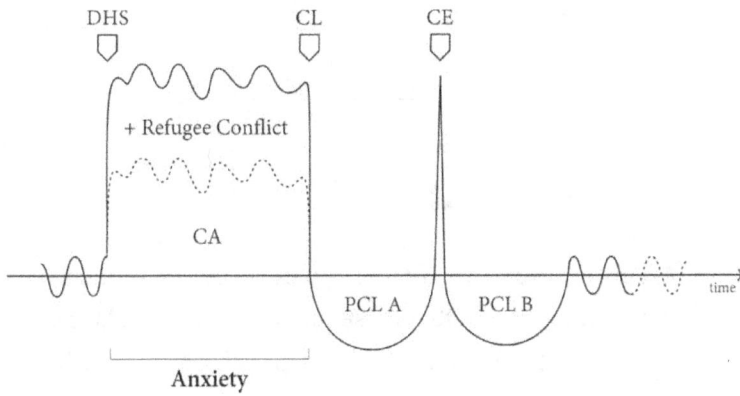

According to the five Biological Laws, all the single demonstrations causing anxiety, they are referable to a certain type of DHS.

If it is true that anxiety is, for the most part, consequent on a certain event that one lives or is living, and it is therefore, easy to correlate it to a precise situation, sometimes, however, the state of anxiety seems not to be connected to something lived, and it induces to define an eventuality of that kind as a "false alarm".

In this case, according to the five Biological Laws, it is possible to explain it with the fact that the person could have taken some tracks (see: cap. Tracks) inducing to activate the biphasic curve previously activated:

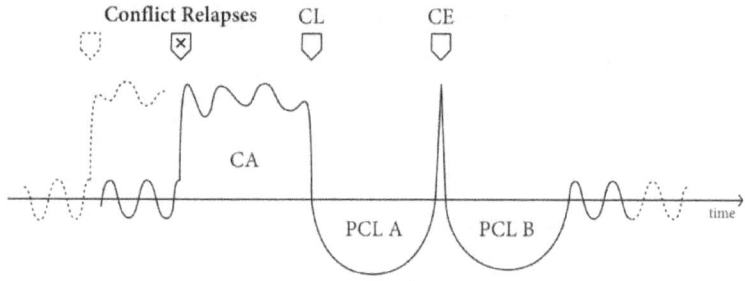

An example can clarify this dynamics better: if one lives a Biological Conflict (DHS) subsequently to a road accident, some tracks, in the instant of the DHS, will fix as: weather in that instant, street or intersection where the accident has happened, season, traffic (line...), dynamics of the accident... afterward, at a distance of a few weeks or month, if some tracks, fixed at the time of the accident, are relived, a reactivation of the native curve (CA) will occur, and anxiety will emerge.

In this case, anxiety represents a "biological alarm bell" to allow the person to react in the best way in such situation, which could be repeated from a biological point of view.

The awareness of what one has lived, it allows to reduce the intensity of the anxiety thanks to the reduction of the Active Refugee.

The Panic Attack

The panic attack are sudden, unforeseen and intense episodes, of a strong state of anxiety, fear and with a rapid escalation of physical and emotional symptoms; they distinguish themselves from all the other forms of anxiety because of the intensity and due to the fact, they are not apparently caused by nothing special. The first panic attack is generally unexpected; it manifests itself "out of the blue".

The most common symptoms, just to mention some of them, can be: palpitations, tachycardia, feeling of suffocation, fear to lose control, to die or go crazy, perspiration, shivers, burst of heat, tremors, chest pain, nausea, feelings of disbandment (dizziness), giddiness, feelings to perceive the external world as unreal…

According to the 5 Biological Laws, and more precisely for the 2° Biological Law, this so acute demonstration, defined panic attack, corresponds to the Epileptoid Crisis:

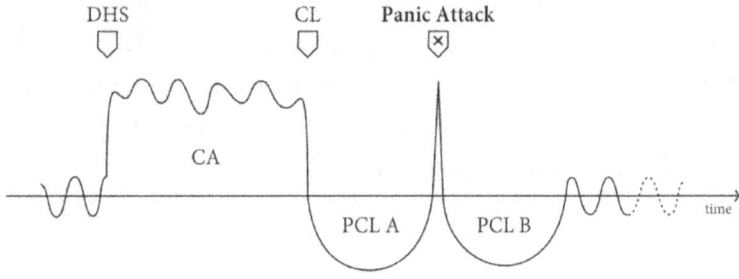

As it is possible to observe by the graph, the Epileptoid Crisis (CE) is preceded by a para-sympathicotonic phase (PCLA) and in effects, who suffers from panic attacks, previously to the attack, he is in a state of calm and comfort both physical and mental, and nothing would make to presage an escalation of so intended neurovegetative demonstrations.

The Epileptoid Crisis represents a sympathicotonic peak that exclusively happens after the Conflict Lysis (CL), and it manifests itself around half of the reparation phase:

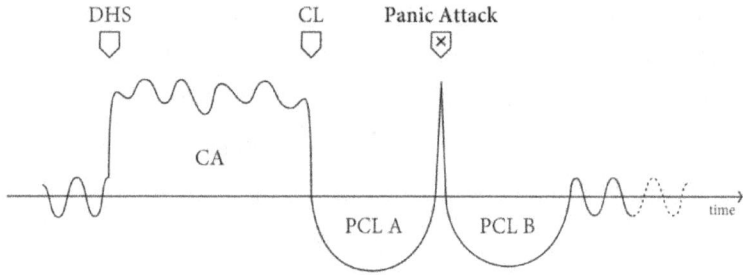

The fundamental function of this ortho-sympathetic stimulation (CE) has the tack to reduce the local edema of the Cerebral Relay (Hamer's focus) activated by the DHS. During the Epileptoid Crisis (Panic attack) one will intensely and acutely relive the same psycho-physical feelings (neurovegetative) that he lived during the DHS.

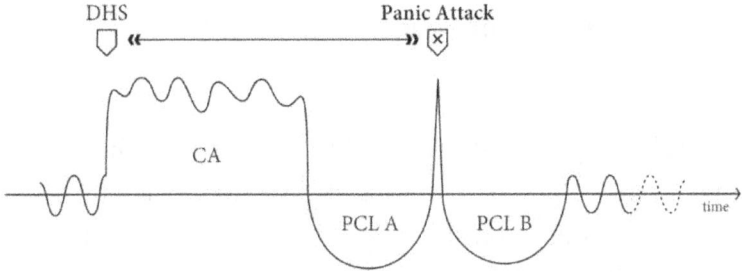

We can understand this way, there is a precise relationship between his own panic attack and an acute event; intense, dramatic (DHS) previously lived. The particularity is that both the Epileptoid Crisis and the DHS have a common denominator, or they are superimposable for what concerns the neurovegetative demonstrations. It is important to understand that between the DHS and the CE some time, days, weeks or more rarely months can go by, and this depends from when the Conflict Lysis happens (CL).

At this point, an example can be clarifying: we hypothesize to have been suffering from panic attacks for about three months and that during the panic attacks, some neurovegetative demonstrations are manifesting as:

- I feel myself suffocating.

- I feel myself forced into a vice.

- I feel some shivers under my skin.

- I feel my legs getting stiff.

- Tachycardia

- Profuse perspiration

- ...

These panic attacks suddenly arrive without any premonitory signal, and they happen when one is in a state of calm, when one is on the sofa, in the car, one is cooking or reading a book...

According to what illustrated, these demonstrations are relative to an activation of the ortho-sympathetic system, and they correspond to the Epileptoid Crisis:

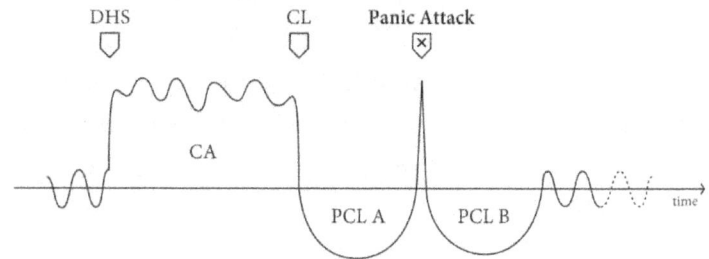

If one has these demonstrations, it means that if one previously lived a situation (DHS) where, decoding the symptoms, one lived an event where he felt himself:

- attacked

- he could not run away.

- ...

Knowing and understanding the five Biological Laws and the course of the biphase curve, it is possible to connect and foresee what neurovegetative demonstrations can be introduced.

It is everything very logical and verifiable by whoever; some people, thanks to personal experience, have reached the same conclusions, but this "personal lived" is "put aside" for the most not finding a comparison in agreement with physicians, psychologists or psycho-therapists.

Summing up the whole speech, we can say that:

The panic attack is a neurovegetative demonstration coming from a biological, acute, intense and dramatic event (DHS) that one previously lived at the first panic attack (CE).

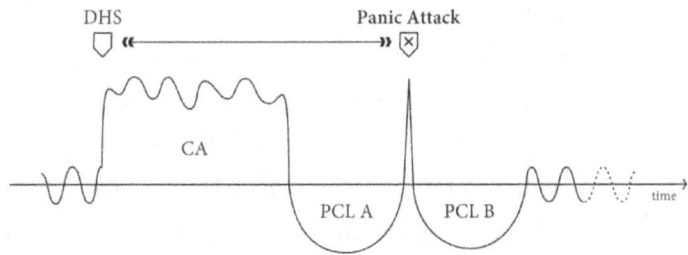

By nature, the course of the biphase curve has a progressive course; a DHS happens; one gets in CA; the CL occurs; one gets in the Post-Conflictlytic phase (PCL), and one CE subsequently happens, just then to return in normotonia;

therefore, one should biologically have a single panic attack; however, this doesn't happen often, but rather continuous panic attacks occur:

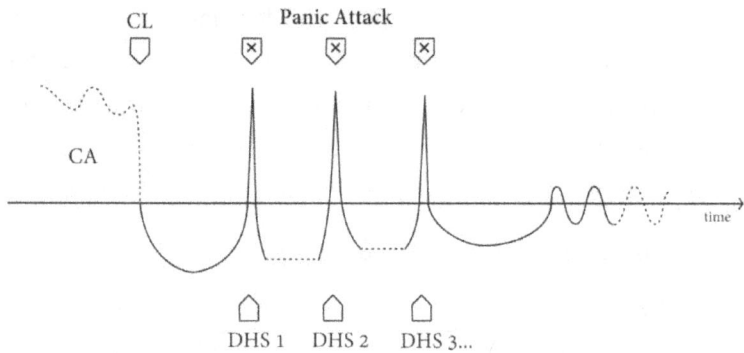

The reason for this course is referable to the fact that when the first panic attack occurs, the person suffers a new DHS in that instant related to his panic attack representing a new DHS because it is an acute event, unexpected, intense he cannot link to nothing in particular. This dynamics besides explaining the reason for which the attacks keep on happening, it also explains the cases in which the panic attacks are modified in the time, they begin with well precise demonstrations and with the passing of time they modify both for that it concerns the type of symptoms and the intensity of the attack.

Continually suffering new DHSs, accordingly new biphase curves and new tracks, which will be maintained in the time, start.

At this point, it can be useful to propose a protocol to try to go back to the origin of our own panic attack.

Before proceeding, it is advisable to have at disposal 20-30 minutes where we won't be disturbed or interrupted for answering to five questions.

Take the whole necessary time and don't be in a hurry to remember, mind needs time to remember.

1. Write here below or on a sheet the date, the most precise possible, in which you have had the first panic attack:

2. Write, not being in a hurry, all the physical and emotional demonstrations that you have during your panic attack (important: if the demonstrations are modified in the time, you should remember and write the first demonstrations of the first panic attacks that you have had):

3. Take some time to remember and enrich of details the physical, psychic and emotional feelings of the panic attack, remember to write everything.

4. Question:

Previously to your first panic attack or to the date that you have marked to the point -1 -, you should have lived a situation in which you felt:

> Read the physical feelings, psychic, emotional that have written at the point -2 over -:

Most probably you succeeded in connecting yourself with the event that has instigated your panic attacks...

If it was not so, you can repeat the protocol how many times you want or can ask yourself a last question:

5. Forgetting for a moment what they have said about your panic attack:

    According to you, what do you trace your panic attacks to?

    To which event? To which situation? To which period?

Close examination

To a following level of close examination and analysis, it is useful to remember that to every DHS it corresponds only one physical a/o psychic symptomatic demonstration, like a key corresponds to a note in the piano.

During a biological shock (event) it is possible to suffer one or more DHSs and consequently, one will have the activation of one or more biphase curves that can have a confused and synchronous course in the time, and every curve will have in itself a lived psychic and an organic correspondence:

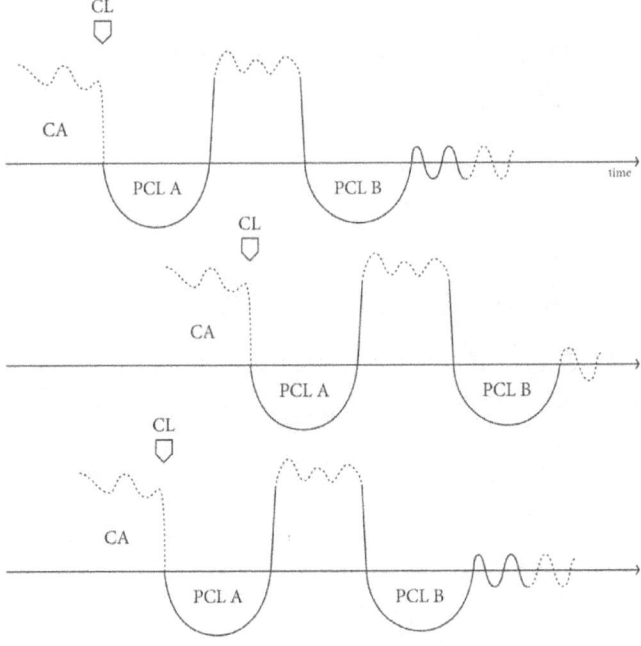

Biologically decoding the demonstrations had during the panic attack, it is possible to go back to the type of lived conflict.

Just to mention some of them, if during the panic attack, it is manifested:

- Difficulty breathing: it means that during the DHS, one lived a conflict of the larynx or the bronchus with the consequent asthmatic constellation.

- Feeling blocked: conflict of the thyroid ducts.

- Feeling to walk on the wadding: conflict of opposition (Beta cells of the Pancreas).

- Feeling to want to break everything: conflict of a grudge of territory (bilious tracts).

- Don't be able to shout: conflict of the larynx (frontal fear).

- Feeling of internal tremor: conflict of feeling attacked (conflict of the derma).

- Muscular tremors: motor conflict (not to be able to escape, to grab,...), the involved muscular group will give greater signs about the lived conflict.

- Intestinal troubles: indigestible contrariety (colon).

- Nausea, vomit: something that one cannot digest (stomach, small bending, cardia).

- Dizziness: checking a situation.

For what concerns the conflicts from the Ectoderm, the Epileptoid Crisis has a duration, for each single attack, of some seconds (10-20 seconds) from the biological point of view, but in practice, often this type of attacks also has a duration of some minutes, and this means that the Epileptoid Crisis turns "in suspension" maintaining for the whole time the sympathicotonic state:

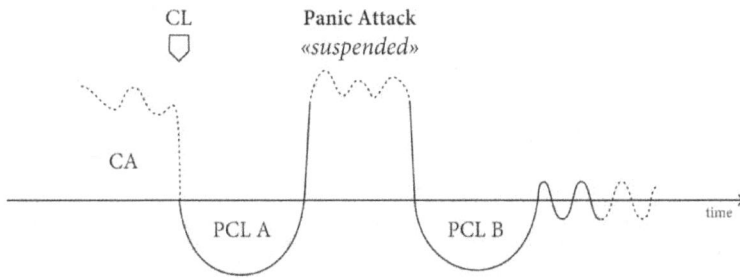

APPENDIX

The Nervous System

The nervous system is anatomically organized as follows:

- **Central Nervous System** (CNS) which comprises the encephalon (brain) and spinal cord (neuraxis): it receives, integrates, and processes the afferent stimuli coming from the Peripheral Nervous System(PNS) which in turn receives the efferent stimuli from the CNS.

- **Peripheral Nervous System** (PNS) consists of cranial nerves and spinal nerves stemming from the spinal cord and it is divided in two main parts:

  - **Somatic Nervous System** (SNS) controlling voluntary responses.

  - **Autonomic Nervous System** (ANS), in charge of involuntary responses, consisting of:

    - **Parasympathetic Nervous System**

    - **Sympathetic Nervous System**

The Autonomic Nervous System, in addition to regulating the homeostasis of the organism, controls all functions of the body that are not normally under conscious control; innervating every tissue, organ and bowel, this system cannot be influenced by will and functions with autonomous mechanisms but still in close mutual collaboration with the Central Nervous System.

The orthosympathetic innervation is traditionally described as a component that performs an escape/attack alert function, mobilizes and organizes energy resources in an emergency or in danger,stimulates the heart and lungs,dilates the bronchi,contracts the arteries and inhibits the digestive system; it prepares the body for physical activity, while the parasympathetic system is a system that allows saving energy, digestion, sleep and rest.

Embryology: the three serous membranes

The embryology is the study of the intrauterine development of the organism from the fertilization (between ovule and sperm) up to the birth. The fertilized ovule (zygote) through some processes of division, differentiation and growth, it will give origin to the fetus. The embryonic development passes through different following phases of segmentation (morula, blastocyst), gastrulation and organ genesis.

In the first three weeks of pregnancy, following the active cellular proliferation, "three populations" of cells (serous membranes) defined: Endoderm, Mesoderm and Ectoderm will be formed.

From these three germinated membranes, for following differentiation, all the tissues of the body will derive. In short and more precisely: from the endoderm, all the tissues forming the alimentary canal and the reproductive system will originate, from the Mesoderm the tissues composing the muscle-skeletal system will originate, and from the Ectoderm the skin, the nervous system, a part of the vascular system will originate…

The fertilized cell (zygote) through processes of division, differentiation and growth will generate the foetus.

Embryonic development goes through several stages of segmentation (morula, blastocysts), gastrulation and organogenesis.

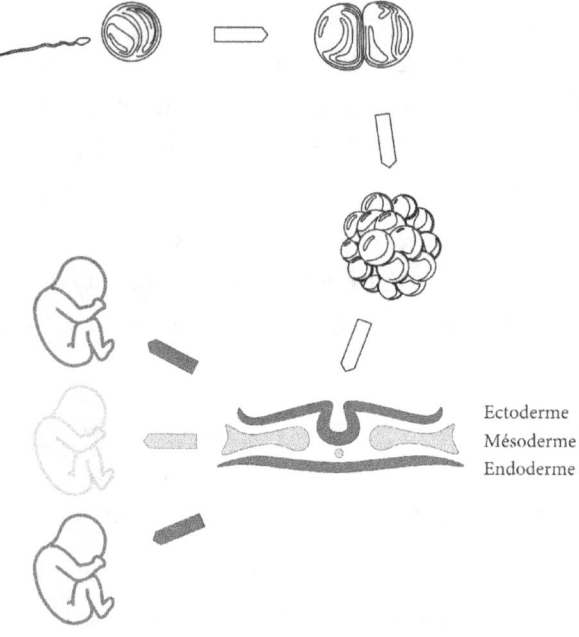

Ectoderme
Mésoderme
Endoderme

In gastrulation, the cells are distributed in three layers of tissue:

- Endoderm
- Mesoderm
- Ectoderm

By subsequent differentiation, all tissues of the body are generated. At the 8th week of gestation, embryonic development is completed to begin organogenesis and the embryo is now called foetus.

CHARTS

The 5 Biological Laws

of **Endodermal origin** tissues

directed by **Cerebral Trunk**

for : "**morsel**" conflicts

Endodermal tissues:

Oral submucosa

Palate

Parotid glands

Sublingual salivary glands

Tonsils

Adenoids *(pharyngeal)*

Lacrimal glands

Iris

Thyroid gland

Posterior pituitary

Middle ear

Eustachian tube

Lower third of the esophagus *(except 2/3 less)*

Alveoli

Greater curvature of the stomach *(except small curvature)*

Liver parenchyma *(except the bile ducts and gallbladder)*

Pancreatic parenchyma *(except pancreatic ducts and Islands of Langerhans)*
Columnar epithelium of the gastro-intestinal
Duodenum *(except the duodenal bulb)*
Small intestine, large intestine and sigma
Inside the navel
Adrenal medulla *(except the adrenal cortex)*
Renal collecting tubules
Rectal submucosa
Trigone of the bladder
Mucosa of the corpus uteri
Bartholin's glands
Fallopian tubes
Ovarian tissue *(except the interstitial tissue)*
Testicular tissue
Prostate
Glands that produce the smegma
Smooth muscle.

The 5 Biological Laws

of **mesodermal** origin tissues

directed by **Cerebellum**

for: **"attack/feeling attacked" conflicts**

Tissues of mesodermal origin:

Derma

Mammary gland (except ducts)

Pericardium

Pleura

Peritoneum

Greater omentum

The 5 Biological Laws

Tissues of **mesodermal** origin

directed by the **White Matter**

for : "self-devaluation" conflicts

Tissues of mesodermal origin:

Connective tissue
Lymphoid tissue *(lymph nodes)*
Tendon tissue
Adipose tissue
Cartilage
Bone
Teeth *(dentin)*
Spleen
Striated muscles
The artery wall
Walls of the veins
Myocardial tissue
Uterine smooth muscle
Muscles of the cervical
Annular sphincter muscles of the neck of the uterus
Muscles *(striated)* of the bladder
Bladder sphincter muscle ring
Smooth muscle of the intestinal tract
Muscles *(striated)* of the rectum
Annular muscles of the anal sphincter

Adrenal cortex

Ovarian interstitial tissue *(excluding parenchyma)*

Testicular interstitial tissue *(excluding parenchyma)*

Renal parenchyma

The 5 Biological Laws

of tissues of **Ectodermal origin**

directed by the **Cerebral Cortex**

for: **"Territorial and separation"** conflicts

Tissues of ectodermal origin:

Epithelium pavimentoso
>   Ducts thyroid
>   Larynx
>   The gill arches
>   The milk ducts(breast)
>   of the bronchial mucosa
>   of the pancreatic ducts
>   of biliary ducts
>   of the renal pelvis and ureters
>   Epidermis
>   of the eyelid and conjunctiva
>   Tear ducts
>   Ducts of the parotid and sublingual glands

Vitreous body, cornea and lens
Tooth enamel
Intima of arteries and coronary veins
Nasal mucosa and paranasal sinuses
Oral mucosa
Mucosa of the upper 2/3of the esophagus
Gastric mucosa(small curvature)

Mucosa of the neck and orifice of the uterus
Vaginal mucosa
Rectal mucosa
Bladder mucosa(excluding the trigone)
Pancreas Cells (alpha and beta)
Periosteum

About the author

Andrea Taddei (Milan 1970, Italy), during the period of his study at the University of Medicine, he learns also different bio-disciplines such as Craniosacral Therapy, Traditional Chinese Medicine, Shiatsu, Ayurvedic Medicine, Yoga and Meditation. Following the abandonment of Academic studies, he devoted full time to the diffusion and study of Craniosacral Therapy. He holds educational seminars and advanced courses on the 5 Biological Laws in Italy and abroad.

The reference site is: www.5biologicallaws.com

Bibliography

English

Dr. Med. Mag. Theol. Ryke Geerd Hamer
Scientific Chart of GNM
Amici di Dirk - Ediciones de la Nueva Medicina S.L.

Andrea Taddei
The 5 Biological Laws and Dr. Hamer's New Medicine
©2012 Andrea Taddei (Sell on Amazon: paperback and ebook)

Andrea Taddei
The 5 Biological Laws: Bones, Muscles and Articulations.
Dr. Hamer's New Medicine
©2013 Andrea Taddei (Sell on Amazon: paperback and ebook)

Andrea Taddei
The 5 Biological Laws: Skin and Allergic Disease
Dr. Hamer's New Medicine
©2014 Andrea Taddei (Sell on Amazon: paperback and ebook)

Andrea Taddei
Craniosacral Network Method
©2014 Andrea Taddei (Sell on Amazon: paperback and ebook)

Spanish

Andrea Taddei
Las 5 Leyes Biológicas y la Nueva Medicina del Doctor Hamer
©2013 Andrea Taddei (Sell on Amazon: paperback and ebook)

Andrea Taddei
Las 5 Leyes Biológicas: Huesos, Musculos y Articulaciones
La Nueva Medicina del Dr. Hamer
©2013 Andrea Taddei (Sell on Amazon: paperback and ebook)

Andrea Taddei
Las 5 Leyes Biológicas: La Piel y las Alergias Cutaneas
La Nueva Medicina del Dr. Hamer
©2013 Andrea Taddei (Sell on Amazon: paperback and ebook)

French

Dr. Med. Mag. Theol. Ryke Geerd Hamer
Tableau scientifique de la Médecine Nouvelle Germanique
Amici di Dirk - Ediciones de la Nueva Medicina S.L.

Andrea Taddei
Les 5 Lois Biologiques et la Médecine Nouvelle du Dr. Hamer
©2012 Andrea Taddei (Sell on Amazon: paperback and ebook)

Andrea Taddei
Les 5 Lois Biologiques: Os, Muscles et Articulations
La Médecine Nouvelle du Dr. Hamer
©2013 Andrea Taddei (Sell on Amazon: paperback and ebook)

German

Dr. Med. Mag. Theol. Ryke Geerd Hamer
Wissenschaftliche Tabelle der GNM
Amici di Dirk - Ediciones de la Nueva Medicina S.L.

Dr. Med. Mag. Theol. Ryke Geerd Hamer
Vermächtnis einer Neuen Medizin, Die "Germanische"
Amici di Dirk - Ediciones de la Nueva Medicina S.L.

Dr. Med. Mag. Theol. Ryke Geerd Hamer
Krebs und alle sogenannten "Krankheiten"- kurze Einführung
Amici di Dirk - Ediciones de la Nueva Medicina S.L.

Dr. Med. Mag. Theol. Ryke Geerd Hamer
Aids die Krankheit, die es gar nicht gibt
Amici di Dirk - Ediciones de la Nueva Medicina S.L.

Dr. Med. Mag. Theol. Ryke Geerd Hamer
"Brustkrebs"- Der häufigste Krebs bei Frauen?
Amici di Dirk - Ediciones de la Nueva Medicina S.L.

Dr. Med. Mag. Theol. Ryke Geerd Hamer
Die Archaischen Melodien
Amici di Dirk - Ediciones de la Nueva Medicina S.L.

Italian

Dr. Med. Mag. Theol. Ryke Geerd Hamer
Testamento per una Nuova Medicina Germanica®
©1999 Amici di Dirk, Ediciones de la Nueva Medicina S.L

Dr. Med. Mag. Theol. Ryke Geerd Hamer
Tabella Scientifica della Nuova Medicina Germanica®
©2007 Amici di Dirk, Ediciones de la Nueva Medicina S.L

Dr. Med. Mag. Theol. Ryke Geerd Hamer
Il Capovolgimento Diagnostico
©2003 Amici di Dirk, Ediciones de la Nueva Medicina S.L

Dr. Med. Mag. Theol. Ryke Geerd Hamer
Il Cancro e tutte le cosidette "malattie"
©2003 Amici di Dirk, Ediciones de la Nueva Medicina S.L

Andrea Taddei
Le 5 Leggi Biologiche e la Nuova Medicina del Dr. Hamer
©2012 Andrea Taddei (Sell on Amazon)

Andrea Taddei
Le 5 Leggi Biologiche: Ossa Muscoli e Articolazioni.
La Nuova Medicina del Dr. Hamer
©2013 Andrea Taddei (Sell on Amazon)

Andrea Taddei
Le 5 Leggi Biologiche: La Pelle e le Allergie Cutanee
La Nuova Medicina del Dr. Hamer
©2014 Andrea Taddei (Sell on Amazon)

Andrea Taddei
Le 5 Leggi Biologiche: Ansia e Attacchi di Panico
La Nuova Medicina del Dr. Hamer
©2015 Andrea Taddei (Sell on Amazon)

Note